Ketogenic
COOKBOOK

Quick And Easy Low-Carb Recipes To Power Through

Christopher J. Lewis

TABLE OF CONTENTS

INTRODUCTION

What was the last endeavor you made at getting thinner of late? Perhaps you took up a serious eating routine program that included just fluids and natural product. Then again you could have picked to do only practice in your neighborhood rec center for a considerable length of time. How did you feel toward the end of this weight reduction administration? Did you figure out how to accomplish the shape you were planning? On the other hand did the eating regimen wind up sounding preferred in principle over practically speaking?

The Ketogenic diet has been changing the lives of every one of the individuals who have chosen to make this idea of eating a piece of their day by day sustenance. Through a novel methodology of high fats, medium protein and low level of starches in your nourishment, the Ketogenic diet demonstrates to you how you can utilize savvy eating with a base measure of activity keeping in mind the end goal to accomplish the weight and state you wellbeing you were searching for. Might you want to know the key to this executioner diet methodology? What are you sitting tight for?

Let's get you started with some fun and quick recipes!

clarifying purposes only and are the owned by the owners themselves, not affiliated with this document.

DISCLAIMER: The purpose of this book is to provide information only. The information, though believed to be entirely accurate, is NOT a substitution for medical, psychological or professional advice, diagnosis or treatment. The author recommends that you seek the advice of your physician or other qualified health care provider to present them with questions you may have regarding any medical condition. Advice from your trusted, professional medical advisor should always supersede information presented in this book.

KETO BREAKFAST MEALS

Peanut Butter Choco Cup

Serves 1-2 people

Calories - 170

Carbs – 10gms

INGREDIENTS

2 Scoops Whey Protein Powder (Chocolate Flavored)

1 ½ Cups Water

½ Cup Heavy Cream

3 Tbsp. Peanut Butter

Ice Cubes (crushed)

METHOD

Blend all the ingredients together till well incorporated. Serve cold.

Morning Protein Fix

Serves: 2

Calories - 163

Carbs: 5gms

Scrambled eggs are a great way to start your day. Here is a yummy recipe for your famished stomachs.

INGREDIENTS

6 eggs

1 cup Mayonnaise

1 ½ Tbsp. Melted Butter

¼ Tsp. Mustard (ground)

1 Large White Onion (Finely chopped)

Salt and pepper, to taste

METHOD

Boil the eggs in a large pot. Once done, let the eggs come to room temperature. Peel the eggs once cooled. Chop them into bite sized pieces and put them in a bowl. Add the remaining ingredients and mix well. Refrigerate till ready to be served / eaten.

Quick Fix Bacon Quiche

Serves: 3

Calories - 290

Carbs: 10gms

This is a classic breakfast dish which is super quick and easy to make and is an absolute treat.

INGREDIENTS

250 gms Bacon Rashers, roughly chopped

10 eggs, whisked

¼ Cup Mozarella Cheese

1 Cup White Onions, Finely Chopped

1 Tbsp Cream

1 Tbsp Oil

1 Tsp. Cayenne Pepper

Salt and Black Pepper, to taste

METHOD

Pre-heat your oven to 375 degrees F. Mix all the ingredients including the cayenne, salt and pepper in a bowl. Whisk the mixture till all the ingredients are easily combined. The cream will add a fluffy texture to the mix. Using a 15 inch muffin tray, drizzle some oil in each section. Pour the egg mix into each muffin section. Bake for 10 minutes till you notice the eggs are cooked.

Serve the quiche warm.

Strawberry & Sage Delight

Serves: 4

Calories – 70

Carbs – 4gms

These fluffy pancakes are really a great inclusion in your Keto diet.

INGREDIENTS

1 ½ Cup Frozen Strawberries

1 Cup Coconut Milk (unsweetened variety)

2 Tbsp. Cream

Handful of Chopped Almonds

1 -2 Sage Leaves

METHOD

In a blender, add all the ingredients and blitz till they are well incorporated.

Serve cold!

Keto Brekkie Hash

Serves: 4

Calories – 150

Carbs – 6.6

INGREDIENTS

1 small onion

1 Zucchini

Pork sausage / Bacon Rashers

1 cup spinach

2 Tablespoons olive oil

2-3 eggs

1 Tbsp. Ghee / Coconut Oil

Salt and pepper, to taste

METHOD

Chop the onions, zucchini and the bacon. In a pan, add the ghee/coconut oil and stir fry the bacon and onions till lightly brown. Add the zucchini to the pan and stir fry for a few more minutes. Fry the eggs separately and place on top of the veggie bacon hash. Serve warm.

Breakfast Meatloaf

Serves: 4

Calories – 190

Carbs – 7gms

Eating meat for Breakfast can keep you energized for a long time and give you all the energy that you need for your daily activities.

INGREDIENTS

12 ounces of pork sausage

1 pound of ground beef

2 cloves of garlic, minced

4 ounces of sliced mushrooms

1 zucchini, chopped

1 Tbspn bacon fat.

1 yellow onion, chopped

2 Tbspns of dried parsley

1 Tspn of garlic powder

2 Tbspns of dried basil

Salt and pepper

METHOD

Take a skillet and place it over medium heat. Add the bacon fat to it. Add the onions and garlic and cook until tender. Add zucchini and place the lid and cook for a few minutes. Add the mushrooms and cover and cook for a few more minutes. Cook until the vegetables have become tender. Add the basil, parsley, garlic powder, salt and pepper and remove the skillet from the heat. Stir well with a spoon and let it remain. After the vegetable mix has cooled down, transfer it to a large bowl. Add the sausage and ground beef and mix it well with your hands. Place the mixture in your crock pot and press down well so that it does not crumple. Cook on low heat for 8-10 hours.

Garnish with avocado and serve.

The Keto Shakshuka

Serves: 4

Calories – 275

Carbs – 7.5gms

Shakshuka is a very popular healthy breakfast dish which is predominantly eaten in North Africa, especially Morocco.

INGREDIENTS

3-4 Eggs, preferably Omega-3 enriched

3 Garlic Cloves

3 Tomatoes

2 Medium or 1 Large Onion

1 Green, Red or Yellow Bell Pepper

Spicy Hot Sauce

1 Tbspn Clarified Butter

1 Cup Water

Salt and Pepper, to taste

METHOD

Finely chop the onions, garlic, tomatoes and bell pepper. Heat a pan and add the clarified butter. Once the butter is heated, add the chopped ingredients to the pan. Toss around till the onions get a transparent color. If you like spice, add paprika or a tspn of your favorite spicy sauce along with salt and pepper.

Add the water to the pan and cover it. Let it simmer for 5-10 minutes. This is the sauce for your shakshuka. Add the eggs on top of the sauce, and cover the pan till you see the egg cooked.

Garnish with chopped Parsley.

Spinach Sausage Stir Fry

Serves – 3 to 4

Calories – 220

Carbs – 5gms

This is a quick and easy breakfast recipe to make, and it is sure to be a hit with the whole family. It can be had for breakfast or for any other meal too.

INGREDIENTS

2 Medium Bell Peppers (Pick any color, red, green or yellow or use 1 of each!)

Handful of Spinach leaves

Chicken Sausages (You can improvise and use any of your favorite sausages)

1 Large Onion

1.5 Tspn Hot Sauce

1 Tbspn Clarified Butter

Fresh Parsley

Salt and Pepper to taste

METHOD

Wash the Spinach leaves under cold water to remove any dirt remaining on it. Roughly, chop the spinach, bell peppers, onions, sausages and parsley. Heat a pan with clarified butter and add all the ingredients to it, beginning with the onions. Add salt and freshly cracked black pepper. Stir for some time. Add your favorite hot sauce to this and let it cook for some time.

Once cooked, garnish with chopped parsley.

Note: You can add any of your favorite vegetables to this dish. E.g., You can even add chopped cabbage.

Avocado Delight

Serves – 2

Calories – 275

Carbs – 10gms

This dish is a creamy combination of avocado and banana along with added nutrition of flax seeds. This smoothie is a great pick me up and hardly takes minutes to prepare.

INGREDIENTS

1 Banana

1-Pitted Avocado

1 Tbspn Flax Seeds

½ Cup Almond Milk (Optional, this is only to be used if you do not like a super thick smoothie)

METHOD

Add all the ingredients to the blender and blitz until you get a puree like consistency. If you feel the smoothie is too thick for you, go ahead and add coconut milk or almond milk.
Serve Cold.

KETO AT LUNCH RECIPES

Spiced Up Chicken Salad

Serves: 2

Calories – 275

Carbs – 5gms

This is a light salad, so if you are at work, you will not be feeling drowsy or lethargic after lunch. You can also make this salad over the weekend and keep in an airtight container. Pour the dressing over it only when you are ready to eat it. You can also chop and add the avocado only when you decide to eat this.

INGREDIENTS
1-Pitted Avocado
1 Mango
2.5 Cups Shredded Grilled Chicken
2 Bowls of Roughly Chopped Lettuce

1 Bowl of Pitted Olives (Black or Green, take your pick)

½ Tbspn Ghee

Paprika

Roasted Cumin Powder

Salt and Pepper to taste

METHOD

Take a pan and add the ghee to it. Once the ghee is heated up, add the shredded chicken to it. Add the paprika and roasted cumin powder and stir-fry for 4-5 minutes. In a bowl or container, add the lettuce, chopped mango, avocado, olives, salt and pepper. Add the Chicken to this mix.

Mix well. Add a dressing of your choice.

Note: If you are not serving or consuming this salad as soon as it is made, avoid adding the mango, avocado and the salad dressing. You could carry the dressing in a little container if you are taking this salad to work.

Cold Green Beans and Walnuts Salad

Serves: 2

Calories – 170

Carbs – 3gms

This quick and easy salad is a perfect summer meal. Light and nutritious, it makes for an excellent lunch especially on days when you are overburdened with work.

INGREDIENTS

2 – 3 Cups Green Beans (Cut each bean into half)

1 Red Onion

½ Cup Walnuts

Salt and Pepper to taste

2 Tbspn Olive Oil

1.5 Tbspn Balsamic Vinegar

METHOD

Chop the Green Beans into 1.5 -2 inch pieces (make it easy to eat). Cut the red onion into quarters. In a pan lightly toast the walnuts, without any oil. Take a large pot of hot salted water, and throw in the green beans. Let them blanch in the pot for 5-8 minutes. The beans should still have their crunch so avoid blanching them for too long.

Remove the green beans and put them in cold water or a bowl of ice cubes to prevent them from cooking further. Mix the salt, pepper, balsamic vinegar and olive oil in a bowl. This is your dressing for the salad. Mix the green beans, onion and walnuts in a bowl.

Pour the dressing over and toss the salad well.

Pan-Fried Chicken With Mango Salsa

Serves: 4

Calories – 290

Carbs – 8gms

The mango salsa adds a nice sweet and tangy touch to the chicken. Makes for a delicious recipe and can be made as a family meal on weekends too.

INGREDIENTS

2 Mangoes

1 Bell Pepper

1 Medium Red Onion

1 Tspn Paprika

½ Cabbage Chopped

½ Cup Freshly squeezed Orange Juice

4 Whole Chicken Legs or Breast or Your choice of cut

2 Tbspn Ghee

Salt and Pepper to taste

Ginger-Garlic Paste

1 Tbspn Balsamic Vinegar

METHOD

Marinate the chicken with balsamic vinegar, ginger-garlic paste, salt, pepper and paprika. Keep in the fridge for 30 minutes. Chop the mangoes, onion, cabbage and bell pepper. To this, add some salt and pepper and the orange juice. Mix well and store in fridge until you are ready to use it. Heat a pan with the ghee. Once hot, add the chicken, leaving it to cook for 4-5 minutes per side. You can baste the chicken with the marinade.

Serve the chicken with the cold salsa.

Chicken Salad

Serves: 3-4

Calories – 300

Carbs – 9.6gms

Here is a delicious cold salad which can be packed and taken to work as well!

INGREDIENTS

1 small chicken, cooked and shredded

2 medium white onions

1 cup mushrooms

Dill, roughly chopped

1 Tbsp. Dijon Mustard

1 Teaspoon olive oil

Eggs (Optional)

Salt and Pepper

METHOD

Mix all the ingredients together and refrigerate.

If you are using eggs, boil the eggs. Once cooled, cut into half. Remove the yoke and mix with the salad. Fill the centre of the eggs with the salad mix.

Low Carb Roast Beef Sandwich

Serves: 2

Calories – 275

Carbs – 4gms

Who doesn't love roast beef! This recipe makes it all the more healthier and delicious.

INGREDIENTS

1 Tbsp Mustard

4-5 Slices Gouda Cheese (Alternatively, you can use cheese slice of your choice)

5-7 Big Lettuce Leaves (depending on the number of sandwiches, increase the quantity)

Roast Beef

Salt and pepper to taste

METHOD

Wash, clean and dry the lettuce leaves. Slice some of the roast beef required. Place the lettuce lead on a plate, then place the roast beef, add on some mustard, salt and pepper and the cheese slice. Fold the lettuce into half or roll the lettuce leaf and dig in!

Beef Chili

Serves: 2

Calories – 270

Carbs – 8gms

INGREDIENTS

1 pound beef meat

1 cup tomato

4 green chilies

1 onion

1 cup olives

1/2 Tablespoon garlic powder

1 Tablespoons chili powder

1/2 Tablespoon smoked paprika

Salt and pepper, to taste

METHOD

First in a wok, cook the beef pieces till it becomes brown. In another pan, add in the finely chopped tomato, onions and olives and sauté it well. Next add in the chilies and the spices. Finally place the beef pieces in the mixture and cook well.

Salmon Sesame Glaze

Serves – 2

Calories – 370

Carbs – 4gms

Salmons coupled with creamy mushrooms make one scrumptious meal.

INGREDIENTS

4 pieces king salmon Fillets

2 ½ Tbsp. Soy Sauce

2 ½ Tbsp. Sesame Oil

3-4 Garlic Cloves (minced)

½ Inch Ginger (Minced)

1 Tbsp. Ketchup (sugar free)

½ Cup White Wine

Salt and Pepper to taste

Parsley leaves

METHOD

In a container, mix all the marinade ingredients. In the same container, place the fish fillets skin side up. Let the fish sit in the marinade for 15 – 20 minutes. In a frying pan, sprinkle sesame oil. Once you notice the pan heated up, place the fillets skin side down on the pan. Cook for 3-5 minutes on each side. Once both sides are cooked, add the remaining marinade to the pan and let the fish boil in it for 2 minutes. Remove the fish from the pan, and add the sugar free ketchup to the sauce in the pan along with the white wine. Let the sauce simmer for 3-4 minutes more and add some freshly chopped coriander.

KETO DINNER RECIPES

Meatballs With Mushroom Sauce

Serves – 2

Calories – 410

Carbs – 7.5gms

This is one of the great Keto recipes that is easy to make and delicious at the same time.

INGREDIENTS REQUIRED FOR MEATBALLS

1 pound veal or beef

½ cup mushrooms

½ onion

¼ Teaspoon dried oregano

¼ Teaspoon dried basil

1 egg

2 Tablespoons parsley

1 Teaspoon raw honey

Salt and pepper, to taste

INGREDIENTS REQUIRED FOR SAUCE

1 Tablespoon olive oil

1 Teaspoon thyme

8 ounces mushrooms

¼ cup red wine

1 cup beef broth

METHOD

In a mixing bowl, add in the chopped onions, eggs, mushrooms and honey. Add in the meat. Next sprinkle the oregano, parsley, and basil and mix well. Preheat your oven to 360 Fahrenheit. Make meatballs which are around 2 inches in size. Place it on a baking sheet. Cook for 30 minutes. While your meatballs are getting ready, you can start making the sauce. For the sauce, take a skillet; add in a little olive oil and sauté the mushrooms for 5 minutes over medium heat. When the meatballs are ready, put them one by one in the sauce. Pour in the beef broth a teaspoon of thyme and allow it to simmer for a few minutes. Pour in the wine and keep stirring till all the flavors have combined.

Seafood Stew

Serves – 2

Calories – 320

Carbs – 4gms

Here is a rich and creamy recipe with lots of crab, fish, prawns and less of work.

INGREDIENTS

1 Pound Mixed Seafood such as Crab meat, fish, prawns etc

1 cup fish stock

½ cup red wine

2 Tablespoons parsley

3 Tablespoons olive oil

15 Tablespoons tomato paste

4 shallots

1 celery stalk

2 bay leaves

2 Teaspoons thyme

Salt and pepper, to taste

METHOD

In a bowl, using a fork break the crabmeat, fish and prawns and mix it well with the parsley. In a pan, pour in some olive oil and sauté it over medium heat for 3 minutes. Pour in the wine and allow it to simmer for 5 minutes. Next on high heat, pour in the fish stock and tomato paste and keep stirring. Make sure to avoid the formation of any lumps. Add in the thyme and bay leaves. Keep stirring and allow it to simmer for 15 minutes. Season it with salt and pepper. Pour sauce over the seafood.

Chicken Kebabs And Eggplant

Serves – 2

Calories – 290

Carbs – 3.9gms

Easy to prepare, delicious to eat with no compromise in the taste, here's a recipe you will try again and again.

INGREDIENTS REQUIRED FOR KEBABS

Skewers

4 chicken pieces

1 onion

1 red pepper

1 green pepper

Olive oil

Salt and pepper to taste

METHOD

In a skillet, pour in the olive oil and over medium heat sauté the onions, green pepper, and red pepper. Add in salt and pepper according to your taste. Dice the chicken pieces. Over medium-low heat, place the chicken pieces on the barbeque. Cook it for 10-15 minutes.

INGREDIENTS REQUIRED FOR EGGPLANT

1 eggplant

2 Tablespoons balsamic vinegar

3 Tablespoons olive oil

2 cloves garlic, minced

Dash of fresh thyme, oregano and basil

Salt and pepper, to taste

METHOD

Slice the eggplants lengthwise in half. In a bowl add the vinegar, olive oil and combine it well. Next mince the garlic, and add thyme, basil and oregano. Brush this mixture on all sides of the eggplant. Place the eggplant over medium-high heat and barbeque it and allow it to cook for 10 minutes on both sides.

Chicken Lasagna

Serves – 2

Calories – 385

Carbs – 6.5gms

Rich and classic lasagna cooked up Keto style!

INGREDIENTS

500g minced chicken

1 onion

1 tomato

3 garlic cloves

2 Tablespoons tomato paste

Dash of sage, basil, thyme, cumin ground

1 Teaspoon cinnamon

1 medium eggplant

2 Tablespoons olive oil

½ cup zucchini

Salt, to taste

METHOD

For the sauce, you need to first sauté the garlic and onion till it is brown. Keep it aside. Next pre-heat your oven to 180 degrees Celsius. Cook the minced meat and keep stirring till they are no big lumps. When the minced meat is well cooked, add in the sautéed onion and garlic into the pan. Mix in the basil, thyme, sage, salt, and cumin according to your taste. Pour in the tomato paste and cook it for 5 minutes. To this add the diced tomatoes and simmer it for 30 minutes. Slice the eggplant and place it at the bottom of your lasagna dish. Layer it with the mince meat mixture. Add a layer of zucchini slices and any other vegetable you like. Pour another layer of minced meat mixture. Bake it in the oven for 30-40 minutes. Leave it to cool for 10 minutes before serving.

Chicken On A Stick!

Serves – 2

Calories – 315

Carbs – 4.2gms

This is a scrumptious meat on the stick recipe you are sure to love.

INGREDIENTS

1 pound chicken breast

1 onion

2 garlic cloves

1 Tablespoon olive oil

¼ cup lemon juice

1 Tablespoon chili flakes

1 Tablespoon ground turmeric

1 Tablespoon ground coriander seeds

1 cup fresh coriander leaves

METHOD

In a food processor blend the garlic cloves, onions, coriander, olive oil, lemon juice, and turmeric till it forms a smooth texture. Dice the chicken into little pieces. Marinate the chicken with the mixture and set aside in the refrigerator for a few hours. Thread the chicken to the skewers and coat it well. Pre-heat your oven to 180 degrees Celsius. Place the chicken skewers on a tray. Line it with baking paper. Bake the chicken in the oven for 30 minutes or until the chicken is cooked well.

Baked Salmon With Herbs

Serves – 2

Calories – 185

Carbs – 4gms

They say that dinner should preferably be the lighter of the meals. This dish will not only satiate your hunger but will also ensure you have a good night's rest.

INGREDIENTS

2 pounds salmon (Ensure the salmon is filleted into thick pieces)

3 Tbspns sesame oil

2 Tbspns light soy sauce

1 teaspoon minced garlic

1/2 teaspoon ground ginger

1/2 teaspoon basil

1 teaspoon oregano leaves

1/4 teaspoon thyme

1/2 teaspoon rosemary

1/4 teaspoon tarragon

½ Cup butter

1/2 cup chopped fresh mushrooms

1/2 cup chopped green onions

METHOD

Stir together the soy sauce, sesame oil and spices and pour over the salmon. Seal it in a bag or a keep it in a box and store in the marinade for 1-4 hours. Preheat oven to 350 degrees F while lining a large baking pan with foil. Lay out fish fillets in a single layer and pour out the marinades into the pan and bake fillets for 10-15 minutes. While the salmon is baking, save time, and get the vegetables ready. Melt the butter. Add the vegetables to it, and mix to coat vegetables. Remove the salmon from the oven, and pour the butter mixture over the salmon fillets, making sure each fillet gets covered. Bake in the oven preheated to 350 degrees F for about 10 minutes more.

Serve warm.

Cabbage Rolls

Serves – 2

Calories – 380

Carbs – 7gms

Easy to make cabbage rolls that you can make any time. You can even make and serve these at parties. This recipe uses chicken mince as a stuffing for the cabbage rolls, however, you can use the meat of your choice, though I prefer beef mince for this recipe.

INGREDIENTS
1 head cabbage
1 pound chicken
1 red onion
2 eggs
1 Teaspoon pepper
1 Teaspoon oregano
1 clove garlic, minced
6 tomatoes

METHOD

Wash the cabbage and remove the leaves. Peel and make a puree of the tomatoes. In a bowl, shred the chicken, add in the oregano, pepper, finely chopped garlic, eggs, and onions and mix it all well. Fill each of the cabbage leaf with chicken mixture and roll it. Place it in a baking dish and pour the tomato puree over it. Cover it with foil. Bake it at 350 degrees Fahrenheit for 30 minutes.

Crunchy Baked Chicken

Serves – 2

Calories – 340

Carbs – 4.8gms

Quick and easy to make, this dish works well when you are back home after a long tiring day at work. You can marinate the chicken and keep in the fridge and pop into the oven whenever you are craving for some comfort food.

INGREDIENTS

1 Cup Almond meal

1 Tspn Paprika

1 Tspn Mustard Powder

½ Tspn Curry Powder

Salt and Pepper to taste

5-6 Chicken Drumsticks

METHOD

Pre-heat your oven to 375 degrees F. Marinate the chicken with the paprika, mustard powder, curry powder, salt and pepper. Keep aside or in the fridge if using later. Put the almond meal in a plate and roll the drumsticks in the almond meal. Take a roasting pan and you can use bacon fat or ghee to grease the pan. Roast for 45 minutes to an hour.

Easy Keto Desserts And Snacks

Kale Crisps

Serves – 2

Calories – 50

Carbs – 10gms

This dish makes for the best healthy finger food instead of the regular packet potato chips.

INGREDIENTS

1 Head Kale, Ribs removed

Sesame Oil

Sea Salt to taste

METHOD

Wash the Kale properly under cold water. Cut the kale into 1-inch pieces. Lay the kale leaves onto a baking sheet and toss generously with Sesame oil and salt. Pre-heat the oven to 275 degrees F. Bake the kale leaves for 20-25 minutes, turning the leaves after every 10 minutes.

Keto Choco Pudding

Serves – 2

Calories – 420

Carbs – 4gms

Indulge yourself in this light and absolutely yum recipe.

INGREDIENTS

1 Cup Cream Cheese

1 Cup Heavy Cream (to be whipped)

1 Bar of Chocolate (90% cocoa) , roughly chopped

Few drops of liquid stevia

METHOD

In a bowl, mix all the ingredients together until they are combined well and smooth. Pour the mix into different serving bowls and refrigerate.

Zucchini Crisps

Serves – 2

Calories – 92

Carbs – 2gms

INGREDIENTS

4 zucchinis

2 teaspoons olive oil

2 teaspoons dry basil

1 teaspoon finely chopped rosemary

Salt and black pepper to taste

METHOD

Preheat oven to 175 °C or 350 °F

Wash and dry the zucchinis and slice them in super thin slices (make sure they are really thin to get extra crispy chips). In a bowl mix the sliced zucchinis with the oil. In another plate mix the rest of the ingredients (rosemary, basil, salt and pepper to taste). Place the zucchinis in a baking sheet (in one layer) and sprinkle with the oregano mix (only one side, don't turn them around). Bake for forty-five minutes or until they are crispy (check every ten minutes to make sure they don't burn)

Note: Let them cool for ten minutes and serve and eat immediately or the chips will lose the crispiness.

Carpaccio Of Shrimp

Serves – 2

Calories – 122

Carbs – 2gms

INGREDIENTS

12 big shrimps

1 tablespoon olive oil

¼ cup finely chopped onion

1 chopped green chili (optional)

1 grated carrot

2 tablespoons finely chopped ginger

1 orange

1 tablespoon lemon juice

Salt and black pepper to taste

METHOD

Wash, peel and devein the shrimps. Fill a pot with water and bring to a boil. Make sure there's enough water to cover the shrimps completely. While the water is boiling, with a sharp knife open the shrimps in half (vertically, making a butterfly shape). Throw the shrimp into the boiling water and bring to a boil again (only for one or two minutes). When you start seeing bubbles in the water remove from heat and drain using a strainer. Put the shrimps on a paper towel so they dry completely while you do the rest of the cooking. Heat the olive oil and stir fry the onions and ginger, remove from heat when they are ready (for about five minutes at medium heat). Squeeze the orange and mix the juice with the lemon juice, season with salt and black pepper to taste. Cut a kitchen plastic bag by half and put it over a cutting board. Place all the shrimps in one layer and cover the shrimps with the other half of the plastic bag. Using a rolling pin flatten the shrimps and then move them to a shallow dish.

Put the ground carrot on the focal point of the dish; sprinkle the shrimps with the green bean stew, the onion panfry and the lemon-orange sauce.

Banana And Apple Fritters

Serves – 2

Calories – 315

Carbs – 9gms

This is a fruity dessert that you can whip up in a few minutes.

INGREDIENTS

2 ripe bananas

1 apple, peeled, cored and grated

1/2 Teaspoon cinnamon

3 Tablespoons coconut oil

METHOD

Mash the bananas in a bowl. Grate apples and mix in with the bananas. To this add in the cinnamon. In a skillet, over medium heat the oil. Drop the mixture on the heated pan and allow it to cook well. Flip it over to cook on the other side. Cook for 10 minutes until it is golden brown at the bottom. Add extra coconut oil if needed.

Coconut-Chocolate Balls

Serves – 2

Calories – 290

Carbs – 12gms

INGREDIENTS

3/4 cup shredded coconut

1 Teaspoon coffee

1/4 Teaspoon salt

1 Teaspoon vanilla extract

1/3 cup macadamia nuts (or nuts of your preference)

METHOD

In a bowl, add in the shredded coconut. Add in the coffee, salt and mix it all well to combine. Next add the vanilla extract. Make sure the mixture is firm. You can refrigerate it for 5 minutes to make it firm. Place the chopped macadamia nuts in a bowl or plate. Make little balls and roll it into macadamia nuts.

CONCLUSION

I do hope you enjoy eating and making these recipes for yourself and your family as much as I did. Nothing is ever difficult as it seems and I have tried to make most of these recipes on a budget. You can even prep for these recipes in advance and have them stored in containers in your fridge.

Good Luck!

FROM THE AUTHOR

If you found this book useful, please take the time to share your thoughts and post a review on Amazon.

It'd be greatly appreciated!

Thank You!

MY OTHER BOOK:

Ketogenic Diet Strategy, Successful Tips & Tricks To Power Through

www.ingramcontent.com/pod-product-compliance
Lightning Source LLC
Chambersburg PA
CBHW070128290526
45789CB00005B/2159